The Psychology Behind Weight Loss

30-Day Challenge

Create Your Mindset

For

Weight Loss Success

Ron Kness

Published by:

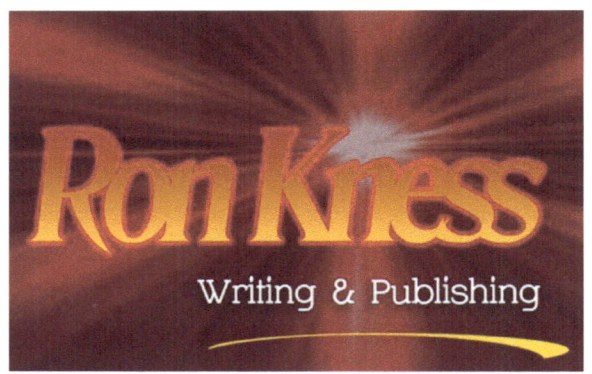

https://ronknesswriting.com

Ron Kness

San Tan Valley, AZ

United States of America

ISBN: 9781070955407

Sneak Peek

A lot of people struggle with weight. According to Health Data, some 160 million Americans are overweight or obese. According to the Centers For Disease Control, 2/3 of American adults are overweight or obese. Those numbers are depressing.

We all gain weight in different ways. Some of us pack on the pounds as we get older, some people gain weight due to a health issue or an injury, while others eat the wrong things. Typically, we diet by eating less. We may exercise more as well, but our weight loss journey revolves entirely around diet and exercise. While that is a big part of weight loss, there is one aspect of it that we overlook. Our thoughts and behaviors play a major role in the challenge.

There are professionals who work with people in order to make changes to lifestyle, behavior, and mindset. People from all walks of life and all ages seek the assistance of psychologists to aid in their weight loss.

Typically, we fall into a pattern of yo-yo dieting. We lose the weight, drop the diet, gain it back, and the cycle repeats itself ad nauseam. In many situations, a primary care physician will refer a patient dealing with a chronic illness or other condition to a psychologist. However, it's something that we could all benefit from because we overlook the importance of mindset in our weight loss journey.

Typically, a psychologist will discuss your goals, medical history, stress level, your social support, as well as your weight loss history. The point is they want to learn about your attitudes toward food and eating, how you view weight loss, what your habits look like, and even get to know your body image.

You might be wondering how that's helpful. Well, did you grow up being told to clean your plate or you wouldn't get dessert? Many of us continue to eat even after we feel full. This is why. We also feel guilty about wasting food when you know that there are people starving in the world.

We have an issue with portion control and then force ourselves to eat it anyway. We are also guilty of eating extra treats because we exercised or coping with stress and boredom by eating.

Your Mindset

All of these common and unhealthy habits are acts of sabotage and they all come down to your mindset.

A positive mindset, one that is pro weight loss will prompt you to make the right decisions, to make healthy choices.

A positive mindset will help gear you toward success. You can do this without the help of a psychologist, of course. However, you cannot dismiss the importance of mindset.

The diet industry is worth billions of dollars. There are countless diets to choose from. Low-carb diets, no-carb diets, low-fat diets, no sugar diets. The food industry supports this by slapping labels on all products. You can see the exact nutritional value of anything and everything that you put in your mouth. It gives you the idea that it's a numbers game, all about math. That's a nice thought, it would be great if it was a simple equation that could be solved. It isn't. Weight loss is rooted in our beliefs, our emotions, and our psychology.

It would be so much simpler if it was a numbers game. You can work out the right number of calories, yes. You can even calculate the right amount of protein, the perfect balance of carbs and fiber, as well as your calorie load. In fact, you might even be wise enough to ensure that each of those meals contains all of the vitamins and nutrients your body needs to thrive, too.

This is what people do when they diet. It's that easy. Except it's not because it doesn't work, does it? If it did, you would be guilty of yo-yo dieting. You can work the numbers as much as you want, but you haven't considered your mindset in your equation. You solved for x but left out a major part of the problem.

PSYCHOLOGY IS 99% OF WEIGHT LOSS

Ultimately, there are three major psychological reasons we fail in our weight loss attempts:

- Stress
- Behavior
- Pleasure

Stress

Stress is one of the biggest factors in our failure to lose weight. It has a direct impact on your journey. Life is busy and when you're trying to cope with a busy schedule, as well as the internal and external stressors of life, it's easy to fall back into unhealthy eating patterns. There is also the presence of the stress hormone cortisol.

Stress causes the presence of this hormone to surge and this triggers survival mode, which means it stores fat, slowing your metabolism down. If you want to lose weight, but you live a stressful life, you have to learn how to manage stress and that is down to mindset.

Pleasure

Pleasure is also one of the keys to weight loss and psychology, all because of its link to stress reduction and management. In order to support weight loss, it's vital that you create a healthy environment, both internally and externally. This will help you manage stress and support the pro weight loss mindset.

That's where pleasure comes in. It's basically a shortcut that will move your body from survival mode into relaxation. It means accessing something that will trigger a relaxation response. You're forcing your body into contentment. These moments provide us with a healthy endorphin release.

Pleasure can also help you remain present when you are enjoying food. When you're present while you eat you are more likely to make the right food choices and stop when you're full.

Behavior

Finally, your behavior. In order to lose weight, you have to adjust your behavior. That means eating healthier foods, drinking more water, working out more often, cutting out unhealthy foods, and so on. So, what is psychological about this when it's literally what "dieting" is? Well, at the foundation of behavior you will find psychology. Your behaviors will be vital to your attempt to build healthy habits, and if you look beneath your behaviors you will find your beliefs, your emotions, and your values.

If you don't truly believe that you will succeed in your weight loss attempts, then how do you think you will solidify a new, healthy behavior? If you believe you deserve unhappiness, you're not likely to take the necessary actions.

We could compile *thousands* of hints and tips to help you on your weight loss journey. However, they will be worthless if you don't adjust your mindset first. Will power is important, but it isn't all about that. It isn't all about ignoring certain foods while embracing others.

Weight loss goes much deeper than that, it's in your psychology.

That's what we are going to challenge you to do over the next 30 days. Before you embark on a weight loss journey, take these 30 days to adjust your mindset to weight loss.

By the way, this 30-Day Challenge is the perfect complement to my book *The Psychology Behind Weight Loss Success*. It is available on Amazon in either Kindle Digital Download (https://www.amazon.com/Psychology-Behind-Weight-Loss-Mindset-ebook/dp/B07SFWVGTY) or hard copy print (https://www.amazon.com/dp/1070768383).

Table of Contents

Legal/Disclaimer Notices

The 30-Day Challenge

Day One – Changing Your Beliefs

If you aren't where you'd like to be, then there's a good chance that your mindset isn't either. Before you go any further, let's touch on what your mindset really means. It's your deeply held beliefs, attitudes, and behaviors that reflect how you perceive yourself, others, and situations. Your mindset influences how you respond as well. Today is the day to change that.

Now, be honest with yourself. What type of baggage are you carrying around when it comes to your weight? It's okay if you don't know specifically, but if you're being truly honest with yourself then you'll have a fairly good idea. You can't change your beliefs until you challenge them and now is the time to do this.

Think about the following statements and ask yourself whether you believe them to be true.

- You come from a family of heavy-set people, it's just the way we're made.
- I've literally tried everything, there's no way I can lose weight.
- There is too much sacrifice required of me to lose weight successfully.
- I just don't have the time to exercise.
- I can't afford to buy the right type of food.
- My <insert condition/injury> won't allow me to exercise properly.
- I'd be more willing to work hard to lose weight if I knew it would definitely work.
- I know how to lose weight; I'll do it when I'm ready.
- Be open and honest with yourself as you consider the statements above. Do they resonate? Don't judge yourself based on your answers, just embrace your newfound awareness.

Day Two – Identifying Your Why

You have probably heard people talk about their why. Do you know what yours is? It's a key part of your journey.

The decision to lose weight may seem like one you make with your rational mind, but in reality, it is one you make with your heart. True lasting motivation always comes from your heart not from your head. A deep heartfelt desire goes a long way to lasting weight loss.

Motivation varies from person to person, it may be a desire to look good, or a more negative one that stems from fear, such as the threat of heart disease or type 2 diabetes that results from overweight and obesity.

Why are you interested in losing weight?

- Are you tired of changing half a dozen times before you feel comfortable leaving the house?
- Are you concerned about your health?
- Do you just want to get in shape?

Make 2 lists as to why you want to undertake this journey. Be honest with yourself. Make a physical list so that you can place it somewhere visible. It could be in your car, on the fridge or even on your bathroom mirror. Take a look at that list before you exercise, look at it before you make dinner. Reference it often. As of now, it's your holy book. Those who have solid motivation and keep in the forefront of their mind for life, enjoy lasting weight loss success.

- Make a list of all the negative consequences of not losing weight
- Make a list of all the positive consequences of losing weight

NEGATIVE CONSEQUENCES OF *NOT* LOSING WEIGHT	POSITIVE CONSEQUENCES OF LOSING WEIGHT

Day Three – Get SMART

Now it's time to create goals. This will help you put yourself in the right mindset. Remember, your goals should be SMART (specific, measurable, achievable, relevant, and time-specific).

Say that your ultimate goal is to lose 100 pounds, you have to be more specific. So, break it down into chunks of 10 pounds or even 5 and set target dates. Think specifically and practically. It's not going to happen overnight, but it's incredibly discouraging when you set unrealistic goals you can't reach.

Another mindset shift that helps in this regard is instead of thinking I need to lose 50 pounds," think "Today, I will focus on changing bad habits, so I will eat a salad for lunch instead of a cheeseburger." One day at a time.

Day Four – Know You're Worth It

This is important:

- Believe you are worth it
- Know *why* you're worth it

Taking a weight loss journey requires sacrifice, energy, money, and time. You have to understand that you are worth it. When you learn to embrace that it makes it easier to maintain your mindset.

Often it is the needs of others that derail your efforts. They need this, they need that, your focus is broken and suddenly, your perspective has been clouded.

Now is the time to write out a list of *why* you're worth this hard work and effort. It's time for you to get to know your value and worth.

Why Am I Worth It?

_____
_____
_____
_____
_____
_____
_____
_____
_____
_____
_____
_____
_____
_____
_____
_____
_____
_____
_____
_____
_____

Day Five – Understanding Your Relationship With Food

What is your relationship with food? Imagine, for a moment, that food is a human being. It's someone that you know well.

Describe your relationship with food.

- What does your relationship with food really look like?
- What does that description look like? Is it a healthy, loving relationship?
- Is it your best friend?
- Your arch nemesis?

_____
_____
_____
_____
_____
_____
_____
_____
_____
_____
_____
_____
_____
_____
_____
_____
_____
_____
_____
_____
_____
_____
_____
_____

Now repeat this exercise, but this time describe junk food as one person and healthy food as another.

_____
_____
_____
_____
_____
_____
_____
_____
_____
_____
_____
_____
_____
_____
_____
_____
_____
_____
_____
_____
_____
_____
_____
_____
_____
_____

Day Six – Accepting Who You Are

Find your favorite mirror in your home and spend five minutes standing in front of it. Now, take a good, long look at yourself.

At this point, you only need to come up with one thing. However, once your time in front of the mirror is complete, you should sit down and make a list of all the things you love about yourself.

What do you *like* about yourself?

_____
_____
_____

_____

_____

_____

_____

_____

_____

_____

_____

_____

_____

_____

_____

This exercise may be painful if you have allowed self-hate to build up within yourself. It's okay if you respond to this exercise in an emotional way. Take a break if need be but come up with a list of at least ten things.

- What makes you a great friend?
- What makes you a good person?

What Make You A Good Friend	What Makes You A Good Person

Day Seven – Visualize Your Goals

It's time to create a vision board. Today, you're simply going to collect all of the images that spoke to you.

You can do this online with a website like Pinterest or create a physical one to hang somewhere in your home. That choice is yours, the purpose of this is to create a visual that truly reflects your goals.

You should choose images that revolve around wellness, weight loss, eating habits, and fitness.

Day Eight – Visualize Your Goals

Now that you have your images, you can put your vision board together.

Remember, there are no limits here – you can put anything you want on it. Once you have completed your vision board, you should invite others to look at it.

Now, this could be sharing it with your family. If you have created a Pinterest board, then you can invite friends to view it. You've visualized your goals, but now it's time to invite accountability.

Day Nine – Gaining Support

It's important that you garner support from the people around you. You have to consider who will offer you appropriate support.

You don't want someone who will respond with judgment, fear or even jealousy. This person (or these people) should be highly supportive.

Think about whom you wanted to share your vision board with, one of those people is your support. This is someone who should help you maintain your positive mindset.

Day Ten – A Love Letter

Today, you should write yourself a love letter.

It's one that you will seal and put away until you achieve your goal. In this letter, you should write about why you decided to undertake this journey, why you feel as though a lifestyle change was necessary.

Think about how you feel about where you are in life. By the time you see this letter again, you will have succeeded in your goal. So, don't forget to mention just how proud you are!

Day Eleven – Investigating Your Triggers

What is it that makes you head to the pantry?

Write it down:

- Think about what triggers your eating.
- What motivates you to eat even when you aren't hungry.
- Is it people?

- Is it certain situations? Are there particular emotions that trigger you?

How can you combat those triggers when you are faced by them? Create a list of actions that will help you combat those emotional issues.

What Triggers Your Eating?	How Will I Combat Those Triggers?

Day Twelve – Find Healing

Are there painful memories lingering within you from your past? Do you struggle to forgive yourself and/or others? This can cause triggers that encourage your unhealthy food habits.

Today, you should take time out to consider what unresolved emotions are swirling around inside of you.

You may determine that you need therapy to help you resolve these issues. However, many of us are completely unaware of those unresolved issues and how they are impacting our lives now. Don't be afraid to reach out for support if you need it.

Day Thirteen – Mindful Eating

Today is your day to be immersed in research.

Look into the idea of mindful eating and find a definition that resonates you. Now, how can you apply the concept of mindful eating to your life? Write it down.

_____
_____
_____
_____
_____
_____
_____
_____
_____
_____
_____
_____
_____
_____

Day Fourteen – You're Beautiful

You are beautiful, and today you need to go out and do something that makes you feel as beautiful as you are.

It might be visiting a department store to have your makeup done, it could be professional photos or a trip to the salon. Whatever it is, go out there and do it.

Day Fifteen – Take Some Time To Relax

This is about you. So, allow yourself to take some time to relax. Treat yourself to a manicure, enjoy time in the backyard with a book, do something, do nothing.

It's all about enjoying an off day. This is your day of self-care.

Day Sixteen – Your Gratitude List

You can keep a gratitude journal if you wish, but for now, let's just focus on creating a list.

- Who do you feel thankful for?
- What things are you grateful for, what about the situations you appreciate?
- Just write out a list of everything you are grateful for.
- Don't underestimate the value of counting your blessings. This is something that can help you bolster your mindset.

People In My Life I'm Grateful For	Things In My Life I'm Grateful For

Day Seventeen – Your List of Positive Affirmations

Do a bit of research into positive affirmations that will support a positive weight loss mindset. Select the ones that resonate with you and write them out.

_____

_____

_____

_____

_____

_____

_____

_____

_____

_____

_____

_____

_____

_____

_____

You should find ten affirmations that speak to you. Take the two most powerful ones and commit them to memory.

You can repeat these when you are struggling. Keep your list handy so you can turn to it when you need it. You may choose to write out a few different lists to keep in different areas.

Day Eighteen – Taking Stock

You want to focus on your health, you want to work on your weight, but first, you have to take stock of where you are in your life.

Look at your family life, career, spiritual self, and social life. How do these things affect your happiness and mindset?

Are you putting too much energy into certain areas while neglecting others? Are there certain people or situations that steal your time and drain your energy?

Write out a list of your priorities.

_____

_____

_____

_____

_____

_____

_____

_____

_____

_____

_____

_____

_____

_____

_____

_____

Day Nineteen – A Healing Ritual

Today is your first attempt at creating a healing ritual.

Once you have yours, you should try to carve out time to practice this once a week. It's simply time for you to focus on healing your body, mind, and soul. Now, this could be a quiet area in your home where you go to pray, meditate or just sit quietly with your own thoughts.

Alternatively, it might be the time you spend journaling or even a hot, bubble bath.

There are plenty of devotionals dedicated to weight loss, you may want to consider investing in one of these. It will simply help you focus and maintain your weight loss mindset.

Day Twenty – Use Music

What type of music do you feel in your soul? What gees you up, makings you feel amazing, and like you could do *anything*? **That is the kind of music you need to incorporate into your daily life.**

You should have an inspirational playlist that helps you boost your spirit and maintain a positive mindset.

There are plenty of streaming services that make creating playlists easy. Make yours and enjoy it as regularly as possible.

Day Twenty-One – Believe It's Possible

Belief is where it all begins really. With belief comes a sense of certainty. You unconsciously believe in your aptitude for success. For example, we can all agree that the sun will absolutely rise tomorrow morning.

We can all agree that gravity will keep us rooted to the ground and that there will be enough oxygen to go around. These are things that we don't actively think about because it is our expectation. Your belief, your expectation should be that you can lose weight. You need a mindset of self-belief.

Where does your belief level sit on a scale of one to ten?

If it's anything less than an eight, then now is the time to work on your belief. Do a bit of research and find some inspirational people to use as a role model. Think about how you will look, how you will, and what it will mean when you have finally achieved your goal weight.

Day Twenty-Two – Step by Step

Inch by inch.

Be honest – what is more important? Your ego or long-term success?

As humans, we often jump in headfirst in order to assuage our egos. You start doing push-ups and your ultimate goal is 100. You can't bear the idea that you can only do five so, you push yourself into doing 100 immediately.

You manage to achieve it, but the following morning you wake up in agony. Your arms are dead weight hanging next to you, your shoulders and triceps burning. It takes you a week to recover.

You're unlikely to go back to the habit and you fail. Instead, you could have started with 20 and worked your way up each day. It is far better to start small and improve slowly and steadily. By doing this you are ensuring your long-term success. By the time you achieve your goal, it is a habit that has become part of your identity. It's just what you do.

This is also true of your eating habits. Small, incremental changes are crucial to long-term success. More importantly, it's easier to maintain a healthy mindset and prepare yourself psychologically when you make smaller changes like giving up cocktails for a month. You're not just conditioning your body; you're conditioning your mind as well.

Day Twenty-Three – It's a Lifestyle

What is crucial to your mindset is to understand that this is not a weight loss diet.

This is a lifestyle you are going to adopt that will help you lose weight, and once you have lost it, will help you maintain it.

If you feel like you must be able to cheat on your goals, then your mindset is all wrong. You're simply setting yourself up to fail.

You have to build a lifestyle that meshes with your identity.

Your new identity is living a healthy life. So, create a bit of interest around your new healthy lifestyle by using special plates to make dinner more interesting. Have a candlelit meal and follow it up with a walk afterward. This is your new normal and you have to accept that.

Consider these shifts in mindset and thinking:

- Learning to feel satisfied with just being satisfied after a meal, and not stuffed
- Learning to identify real hunger versus a mental desire to eat (for other reasons)
- Being able to overcome cravings
- The ability to monitor food intake – which includes mindful eating and portion control
- Develop healthy coping skills for stress, and negative emotions
- Be comfortable with and accept that food restrictions and portion sizes are a natural part of a healthy weight
- Accept that lasting habit changes are needed for lasting weight loss and this means that healthy thinking must be maintained for life

Day Twenty-Four – Modifying Behaviors & Thoughts

One of the most important aspects of your weight loss journey is reinforcing your healthy thoughts and behaviors. Often, we allow old thoughts to resurface. The process of weight loss often feels like a punishment so, it's easy to slip back into old habits.

Create a list of healthy rewards to reinforce the positive thought, behavioral modifications that you make, and milestones of weight lost you reach. Food is not a reward, remember that.

_____
_____
_____
_____
_____
_____
_____
_____
_____
_____
_____
_____
_____
_____
_____
_____
_____

Day Twenty-Five – Change of Heart, Change of Mind

Obviously, we have focused on mindset. That's what we're dealing with. It's all about adjusting your mindset. However, it would be remiss to go through this 30-day challenge without also encouraging you to think about your heart.

While your mindset is key to maintaining your motivation and attitude throughout your weight loss journey, you also need a change of heart. It's likely your heart that kicked all of this off after all. Your heart pushed you to this point so you should thank it for getting you this far.

More importantly, remember that it started your motivation and take a moment to write out why that was.

_____
_____
_____
_____
_____
_____
_____
_____
_____
_____
_____
_____
_____
_____
_____
_____

Day Twenty-Six – Exercise Self-Discipline

It's like a muscle, it needs to be strengthened which means you need to exercise it regularly. **Go out of your way to exercise your self-discipline today.**

Day Twenty-Seven – Elimination

Now you can put your self-discipline into action. Today, reduce your consumption of a food or beverage that you know is bad for you.

If you're a big soda drinker, then cut back. If coffee is your guilty pleasure, reduce your intake by a cup. If you can't get through a day without eating two candy bars, cut it down to one. This is your opportunity to exercise your self-discipline and test your mindset.

Day Twenty-Eight – History is Your Teacher

History is your teacher; it should never be your jailer. We already touched on forgiving yourself for your past and moving forward with the lessons that you've learned.

It's time to revisit the exercise of day twelve.

- Have you truly started healing from past pain?
- It's been two weeks since you thought about those situations and events. How do you feel about them now?
- Have you been able to make progress on controlling emotional triggers? If not, how will you do so going forward?

_____
_____
_____
_____
_____
_____
_____
_____
_____
_____
_____
_____
_____
_____
_____
_____

Day Twenty-Nine – Food Associations

Remember, your behaviors are simply learned habits. We tend to associate certain activities, experiences, and emotions with a particular set of behaviors.

For example, if you sit down to watch an hour of television every night and you do so with a pint of ice cream, then your brain is making an association between the two. Often, you're not even hungry.

However, your brain has synced the two activities into one. You sit down to watch television and your brain urges you to eat. That's why it's so difficult to snap yourself out of these habits.

Today, consider what your brain associates with food. Your brain will convince you that you're hungry when you sit down to watch television.

So, to help break the association you can start by enjoying a healthy snack at that time. Carrot sticks are a good option since they have a satisfying crunch and a touch of sweetness to them. If you don't *want* carrot sticks, then you're probably not hungry. Just enjoy your show.

Day Thirty – Emotion Identification

We've already touched on the emotions that are linked to overeating. Let's come back to it. When you feel like overeating or eating the wrong foods, what are you feeling?

Think long and hard about what prompts you to walk to the cupboard or vending machine to get a hit of junk food.

- Are you bored?
- Do you feel stressed out?
- Are you exhausted?
- Do you feel sad?

It could be a combination of these things.

_____
_____
_____
_____
_____
_____
_____
_____
_____
_____
_____
_____

The point is that oftentimes, you aren't hungry when you experience these triggers so, you have to find another way in which you can meet that emotional need. That's your exercise for today.

Remember, your brain will perceive these changes as a threat. So, it will actively attempt to trick you and justify your bad decision. That's why your mindset is so important. You must be strong enough to resist and maintain your focus on your weight loss journey.

About the Author

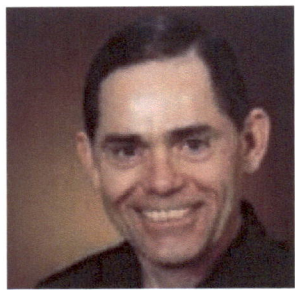

I have published numerous books on Amazon for Kindle, Draft2Digital. Lulu and other publishing platforms, both in electronic and POD formats.

While most of my books are on health and fitness in general, my topics of interest are leaning more toward aging baby boomers and the older population and the health and fitness issues they face.

Besides my own writing, I also ghostwrite ebooks, books, reports, articles, blogs and do Kindle conversions for clients on a variety of topics. Go to my website at http://ronknesswriting.com for more information or to submit a quote. For a complete list of my books, go to https://www.amazon.com/Ron-Kness/e/B0072M6PYO.

Today my wife and I are retired from our careers and live in San Tan Valley, AZ. I now write as a retirement business where you'll find me happily sitting in my office typing away on my laptop as I work on my next book or ghostwriting project . . . that is if we are not traveling on a cruise ship - our new-found mode of travel.

www.ingramcontent.com/pod-product-compliance
Lightning Source LLC
Chambersburg PA
CBHW060808290526

45792CB00005BA/1565